NAVIGATING UTERINE CANCER WITH CONFIDENCE AND CARE

Transformative Strategies For Cancer Recovery For Better Reproductive Health And Fertility

DR. WESLEY IAN

DISCLAIMER

The information in this book is not meant to replace professional medical advice, diagnosis, or treatment; rather, it is meant mainly for general informational reasons. If you have any questions about a medical problem, you should always consult your doctor or another trained health expert. Don't ever discount expert medical advice or put off getting it because of something you've read in this book.

Any negative effects or repercussions arising from the usage of the material provided herein are not the responsibility of the book's author or publisher. It should be noted by readers that the material in this book is not all-inclusive and might not address every facet of the subject. Furthermore, new research may have an impact on how health concerns are understood or treated because medical knowledge is always changing.

No particular test, treatment, method, or product mentioned in this book is endorsed or promoted by the author or publisher. The reader assumes all risk associated with using the information included in this book.

Before making any big decisions regarding your health, it's crucial to speak with a licensed healthcare provider. The relationship between a patient and their healthcare practitioner should not be replaced by this book, nor is it meant to offer medical advice.

The opinions presented in this book are the author's and may not necessarily represent those of the publisher. Any errors, omissions, or inaccuracies in the information in this book are not the responsibility of the author or publisher.

It is recommended that readers independently confirm any information contained in this book and speak with a healthcare provider about their specific medical needs and state of health.

TABLE OF CONTENTS

ABOUT THE BOOK

"Navigating Uterine Cancer with Confidence and Care" is an extensive manual that is an essential tool for people dealing with uterine cancer. An insightful preface welcomes readers and expresses thanks at the start of the book. It explains the goal of the book and emphasizes how important it is to confront uterine cancer with care and confidence, laying the groundwork for an inspiring journey.

With a focus on the disease's basic features, it gives readers a comprehensive grasp of uterine cancer, including its kinds, risk factors, and diagnostic procedures. Those who possess this fundamental understanding are better able to make educated decisions when they travel.

"Empowering Yourself with Knowledge," highlights how knowledge can change how you approach uterine cancer. It gives readers research tips for their diagnosis and equips them with the knowledge and skills they need to communicate with their healthcare provider and get second opinions.

The book examines the significance of creating a strong support system in light of the need for emotional support. The chapter covers the holistic requirements of people dealing with uterine cancer, from joining support groups and seeking professional counseling to efficiently communicating with family and friends.

It turns into a crucial tool for navigating the possibilities for treatment and making decisions. By giving readers a comprehensive understanding of various therapies such as immunotherapy, hormone therapy, chemotherapy, radiation therapy, and surgery, they may make educated decisions about their care.

The management of side effects from treatment and preserving general well-being during the journey is the focus. These chapters provide helpful advice for overcoming the difficulties of therapy, from comprehending typical side effects to investigating integrative therapies and stressing the significance of diet and wellness.

"Life After Treatment," provides information on follow-up care, survivability, and coping mechanisms for recurrence anxiety. It honors achievements and offers a road map for people moving from active treatment into a post-treatment life.

The book goes into additional detail about the particular issues of fertility and reproductive health. It explores preservation choices, coping techniques for handling changes in reproductive health, and the effect of uterine cancer on fertility.

The book concludes by promoting awareness and self-empowerment. It inspires people to take on the role of their advocates, spread the word about uterine cancer, and actively support advancements in the field of uterine cancer research.

"Navigating Uterine Cancer with Confidence and Care" essentially goes above what is typically expected of a medical manual. It provides information on uterine cancer while also supporting the reader's emotional health and encouraging a holistic approach to overcoming the obstacles presented by this diagnosis.

CHAPTER ONE

INTRODUCTION TO UTERINE CANCER

COMPREHENDING CERVICAL CANCER

One of the most common gynecological cancers, uterine cancer, is a major global health concern for women. An essential part of the female reproductive system, the uterus, experiences aberrant and unregulated cell proliferation in this illness.

To have a thorough understanding of uterine cancer, it is necessary to examine several topics, such as its definition, kinds, risk factors, symptoms, and the diagnostic techniques used to identify and stage the disease.

UTERINE CANCER: WHAT IS IT?

The uterine lining, or endometrium, is where uterine cancer, commonly referred to as endometrial cancer, begins. In the female reproductive system, the uterus is essential because it houses and nurtures a fertilized egg during pregnancy.

This complex mechanism is upset by uterine cancer, which causes the endometrium's cells to proliferate abnormally. Examining the variables that influence the growth of uterine cancer as well as the complex interactions between biological processes that result in its appearance is necessary to comprehend the nature of this disease.

UTERINE CANCER TYPES

It is important to note that uterine cancer is not a single illness, but rather a group of subtypes with varying traits and target cells. Endometrial carcinoma, which develops from the cells lining the uterus, is the most prevalent type. Uterine sarcoma is another less common but more dangerous form that starts in the uterus's muscles or other tissues. Since various types may react differently to therapeutic interventions, these distinctions are essential in choosing the best course of action.

RISK ELEMENTS AND ORIGINS

It is crucial to comprehend the causes and risk factors of uterine cancer to prevent the disease and diagnose it early. Age, obesity, hormonal imbalances, and medical history of certain illnesses including diabetes and polycystic ovarian syndrome (PCOS) are among the factors that raise the risk. Furthermore, the risk can be increased by exposure to estrogen in the absence of progesterone's balancing effects, as in the case of hormone replacement therapy (HRT). A family history of colorectal or uterine cancer is one example of a genetic component that contributes to the complex interaction between genetics and environment.

SYMPTOMS AND INDICATIONS

Early detection and treatment of uterine cancer depend critically on the ability to identify its warning signs and symptoms. The main symptom is abnormal vaginal bleeding, particularly postmenopausal bleeding. Changes in bowel or urine habits, inexplicable weight loss, and pelvic pain or discomfort are possible additional indications. Although these symptoms are not exclusive to uterine cancer, their existence calls for immediate medical intervention to rule out other possible illnesses and start treatment as soon as possible.

RECOGNITION AND SEQUENCING

The path to a uterine cancer diagnosis is a methodical process to verify the existence of cancer and estimate its spread. To obtain tissue samples for analysis, typical diagnostic techniques include dilatation and curettage (D&C), endometrial biopsy, and transvaginal ultrasonography. After a diagnosis, staging is essential for determining whether the disease has progressed outside of the uterus. By assessing the degree of invasion, lymph node involvement, and possible metastasis, staging helps medical practitioners create a treatment plan that is suitable for the patient's condition.

CHAPTER TWO

TAKING CONTROL OF YOURSELF VIA KNOWLEDGE

THE INFORMATION GAP IN THE BATTLE AGAINST UTERINE CANCER

Gaining knowledge is essential for negotiating the complexities of medical conditions, particularly when dealing with a disease as serious as uterine cancer. Comprehending the significance of knowledge in the context of uterine cancer is vital since it forms the basis for making well-informed decisions regarding one's health. Information is a potent instrument that gives people the knowledge and understanding needed to take an active role in their healthcare journey.

INVESTIGATING YOUR PROGNOSIS

It is crucial to conduct an in-depth study on uterine cancer after receiving a diagnosis. You can have a better grasp of uterine cancer's characteristics, phases, available treatments, and possible adverse effects by researching your diagnosis. This information not only makes people feel more empowered, but it also makes it possible for them to interact with healthcare professionals more successfully.

Well-informed patients are better able to actively engage in discussions regarding their treatment plans and make choices that are consistent with their values and preferences.

QUESTIONS TO PUT TO YOUR MEDICAL STAFF

During the information-gathering phase, it is critical to develop pertinent questions to pose to your healthcare staff. This proactive approach guarantees that no detail of your diagnosis or treatment plan is left unclear, while also facilitating effective communication.

The details of the diagnosis and the advantages and disadvantages of various treatment choices are just a few examples of the questions that may come up. Establishing a collaborative connection with your healthcare team through open and honest communication allows both sides to participate in the decision-making process.

LOOKING FOR SECOND OPINIONS

Getting second views is another essential component of self-determination when dealing with uterine cancer. It is evidence of the proactive approach people might take when seeking treatment. Getting a second opinion might provide fresh viewpoints, new information, and even different approaches to therapy.

This phase gives confidence in the selected course of action and gives a more thorough grasp of the diagnosis. Getting a second opinion is a responsible and knowledgeable way to make sure you get the best possible result, not a show of mistrust.

Accepting information as a guiding force is essential to arming yourself with knowledge in the face of uterine cancer. Important steps in this empowering process include researching your condition, creating appropriate questions for your healthcare staff, and getting second views.

Through active involvement in your healthcare journey, you will not only gain a deeper awareness of uterine cancer but will also be part of the team working to find the most efficient and customized course of treatment.

CHAPTER THREE

CREATING A SUPPORT NETWORK

THE VALUE OF PSYCHOLOGICAL ASSISTANCE

Creating a strong support network is crucial for overcoming obstacles in life and advancing general well-being. Emotional support is one of the main pillars of this support system and is essential for developing both mental and emotional resilience. Providing empathy, comprehension, and compassion as well as establishing a safe space where people can express their thoughts and feelings without fear of repercussions are all components of emotional support. This type of support reinforces the impression that people are not alone in their challenges and acts as a buffer against stress, worry, and loneliness.

SPEAKING WITH FRIENDS AND FAMILY

Keeping in touch with loved ones and friends is another essential component of creating a robust support system. These connections, which are based on mutual familiarity and history, provide a feeling of acceptance and unwavering love. Within these relationships, good communication facilitates problem-solving as well as the sharing of victories and joys. Honest and open communication improves relationships and makes it possible for loved ones to offer insightful opinions, counsel, and support. People feel understood and supported in this environment because of the camaraderie these talks establish.

TAKING PART IN SUPPORT GROUPS

Getting involved in support groups offers a special way to meet people who have gone through similar struggles and experiences. Support groups provide a forum for people to share advice, coping mechanisms, and encouragement, regardless of whether they are dealing with a particular medical condition, life transition, or personal challenge. These groups' common understanding lessens stigma and feelings of isolation, fostering a caring environment where members may share knowledge and feel empowered.

EXPERT GUIDANCE AND THERAPY

Getting professional counseling and treatment is essential to enhancing one's network of support. Professionals with training, including therapists and counselors, provide specific direction and assistance based on each person's requirements. These experts offer a private setting where people can explore their feelings and ideas, create coping strategies, and learn more about themselves. With its insights and methods that support general well-being, therapy is a useful tool for resolving mental health challenges, interpersonal issues, and personal growth.

Creating a support network entails appreciating the value of emotional support, encouraging candid conversations with loved ones, looking into support groups, and, if necessary, obtaining professional counseling. These interdependent components form a complex web that supports mental health, builds resilience, and facilitates a happy and well-supported life journey.

CHAPTER FOUR

OPTIONS FOR TREATMENT AND MAKING DECISIONS

SURGERY

The lining of the uterus is where uterine cancer, sometimes referred to as endometrial cancer, first appears. Numerous factors, such as the patient's general health, personal preferences, and the cancer stage, influence the treatment choices available for uterine cancer. When deciding on the best course of action, patients and healthcare professionals alike must have a thorough awareness of different therapeutic approaches.

The mainstay of treatment for uterine cancer is surgery, which comes in many forms and involves different factors. The most frequent surgical procedure is a hysterectomy, which entails the uterus being removed. Additional treatments such as lymph node dissection or tissue excision from the surrounding area can be required, depending on how far the cancer has gone.

Minimally invasive surgical methods such as laparoscopy are also available; these methods provide shorter recovery periods and less pain throughout the procedure.

RADIATION THERAPY

Another essential part of the treatment for uterine cancer is radiation therapy. High-energy radiation is used to target and eliminate cancer cells. Common methods include external beam radiation and brachytherapy, which involves placing a radioactive source inside or close to the tumor. Depending on the particulars of the cancer, radiation therapy may be used as the only treatment or in addition to surgery and chemotherapy.

During chemotherapy, medications are used to either kill or stop the growth of cancer cells. Targeting cancer cells that have perhaps spread outside of the uterus, this systemic medication flows throughout the body. When uterine cancer is in an advanced stage or there is a high chance of recurrence, chemotherapy is frequently advised. Healthcare professionals collaborate closely with patients to manage the various side effects of chemotherapy and improve their overall quality of life while undergoing treatment.

HORMONE TREATMENT

When a malignancy is sensitive to hormones like estrogen, hormone therapy is used. Hormone treatment tries to stop the proliferation of cancer cells by either preventing the generation of estrogen or interfering with its function. Certain uterine tumors, especially those with hormone receptors, are more frequently treated with this method.

A relatively new area of cancer treatment called immunotherapy works by encouraging the body's immune system to seek out and destroy cancerous cells. Immunotherapy is still being studied for uterine cancer, but in some cases, the results are encouraging.

It may be considered as part of a comprehensive treatment strategy or as part of clinical trials examining its efficacy in uterine cancer care.

Making informed treatment options is a vital element of uterine cancer therapy. Patients and healthcare providers collaborate to weigh the benefits and potential risks of each treatment option, taking into account the individual's health, preferences, and the specific characteristics of the cancer. Factors such as age, overall health status, and potential impact on fertility are essential considerations in the decision-making process. Open communication between the patient and the healthcare team is key, fostering a shared decision-making approach that aligns with the patient's values and goals for treatment outcomes. Educational resources, support networks, and second opinions may also play crucial roles in enhancing the decision-making process, ensuring that the chosen treatment plan is well-informed and aligned with the best interests of the patient.

CHAPTER FIVE

MANAGING TREATMENT SIDE EFFECTS

UNDERSTANDING COMMON SIDE EFFECTS

When embarking on a course of medical treatment, it is crucial to be well-informed about the potential side effects that may accompany the prescribed interventions. Understanding common side effects enables patients to anticipate and manage these challenges effectively.

Healthcare providers play a pivotal role in educating patients about the expected adverse reactions associated with specific treatments, fostering a proactive approach to side effect management. By acknowledging and comprehending common side effects, individuals are better equipped to make informed decisions regarding their care and to engage in open communication with their healthcare team.

NAVIGATING PHYSICAL CHANGES

The physical changes that often accompany medical treatments can significantly impact an individual's quality of life. Managing physical changes requires a multifaceted approach that addresses both the immediate symptoms and their broader implications. For instance, changes in appearance, such as hair loss or weight fluctuations, may necessitate adjustments in daily routines and self-perception. Healthcare providers should offer practical guidance on coping strategies, from the use of supportive devices to lifestyle modifications. Moreover, fostering a supportive environment and encouraging open dialogue about physical changes can empower individuals to adapt and maintain a sense of control over their bodies during treatment.

EMOTIONAL AND PSYCHOLOGICAL WELL-BEING

The emotional and psychological toll of medical treatments and their associated side effects should not be underestimated. Patients often grapple with anxiety, depression, and stress, which can arise from the uncertainty of their health status and the challenges posed by treatment regimens. A holistic approach to healthcare includes addressing the emotional and psychological well-being of individuals undergoing treatment. Mental health support, counseling services, and peer support groups can provide invaluable resources for patients to express their feelings, share experiences, and receive guidance on coping mechanisms. Recognizing the interconnectedness of physical and mental health is essential in fostering a comprehensive and patient-centered approach to care.

INTEGRATIVE THERAPIES AND COMPLEMENTARY MEDICINE

In the realm of managing treatment side effects, integrative therapies and complementary medicine play a vital role in enhancing overall well-being. These approaches encompass a range of practices, such as acupuncture, yoga, massage, and dietary supplements, which can complement conventional medical treatments. Integrative therapies aim to address the physical, emotional, and spiritual aspects of health, offering patients additional tools for symptom management and overall comfort. While these practices may not replace conventional medical interventions, they can serve as valuable adjuncts, promoting a holistic approach to healthcare. Collaborative discussions between healthcare providers and patients about the integration of complementary therapies can contribute to personalized and patient-centered care plans.

CHAPTER SIX

NUTRITION AND WELLNESS DURING TREATMENT

IMPORTANCE OF NUTRITION

Nutrition plays a crucial role in supporting overall health, particularly during times of medical treatment. The importance of nutrition cannot be overstated, as it directly influences the body's ability to heal, recover, and maintain optimal functioning. Adequate nutrition provides essential nutrients that contribute to immune system strength, tissue repair, and energy levels. For individuals undergoing treatment, a well-balanced diet becomes even more critical, as it aids in mitigating potential side effects, supporting medication effectiveness, and promoting a sense of well-being.

DIETARY CONSIDERATIONS

Dietary considerations become paramount during treatment, requiring a personalized approach based on the specific medical condition, treatment plan, and individual needs. It is essential to address potential nutrient deficiencies that may arise due to the treatment itself or side effects such as nausea, loss of appetite, or changes in taste. Tailoring the diet to include nutrient-dense foods, and supplements if necessary, and adapting to individual preferences helps ensure that nutritional goals are met. Collaborating with healthcare professionals, including dietitians, can provide valuable guidance in creating a dietary plan that aligns with treatment objectives.

PHYSICAL ACTIVITY AND EXERCISE

Physical activity and exercise also play a vital role in the overall wellness of individuals undergoing treatment. While the level of physical activity may need to be adjusted based on the individual's health status and treatment protocol, incorporating gentle exercises such as walking, stretching, or yoga can contribute to improved mood, energy levels, and overall quality of life. Exercise has been shown to enhance the effectiveness of certain treatments, alleviate treatment-related fatigue, and support cardiovascular health.

Engaging in physical activity should be approached with moderation and consultation with healthcare providers to ensure safety and appropriateness.

TECHNIQUES FOR STRESS MANAGEMENT

Stress management techniques are integral components of a comprehensive approach to wellness during treatment. The emotional and psychological aspects of coping with a medical condition can significantly impact overall well-being. Various stress management strategies, such as mindfulness meditation, deep breathing exercises, and relaxation techniques, can help individuals navigate the emotional challenges associated with treatment. These practices not only promote mental health but also contribute to better physical outcomes by reducing stress-related inflammation and supporting the body's natural healing processes.

A holistic approach to nutrition and wellness during treatment encompasses the importance of a well-balanced diet, personalized dietary considerations, appropriate physical activity, and effective stress management techniques. This multifaceted approach not only addresses the physiological aspects of health but also considers the emotional and psychological well-being of individuals undergoing treatment. Collaborating with healthcare professionals to tailor strategies to individual needs ensures a comprehensive and supportive approach to navigating the challenges associated with medical treatment.

CHAPTER SEVEN
LIFE FOLLOWING THERAPY
SURVIVORSHIP AND CONTINUED CARE

For cancer survivors, life after treatment is the start of a new chapter known as survivorship. The era of survival has its own set of difficulties and adaptations. Even though the end of treatment is unquestionably a big step forward, medical care doesn't end there. Survivorship care entails periodic evaluations and follow-up visits to track the patient's health and handle any possible problems that might develop after treatment. Tracking the survivor's development, spotting any recurrence signals, and managing the long-term effects of cancer and its therapy all depend on these follow-up appointments.

KEEPING AN EYE ON YOUR HEALTH

Following cancer treatment, it's critical to keep a close check on one's health. A crucial part of post-treatment monitoring is routine physical examinations, screenings, and diagnostic testing. These assessments enable prompt response and aid in the early identification of any possible problems. Monitoring health encompasses not only physical examinations but also evaluations of mental and emotional well-being.

To manage chronic diseases, address any lasting side effects, and maintain general health and vitality, survivors may collaborate closely with medical practitioners.

HANDLING THE FEAR OF RECURRENCE

Among cancer survivors, fear of recurrence is a common and natural concern. The dread of the disease returning can be a persistent emotional challenge during the shift from active therapy to the post-treatment phase. To control this dread and keep it from overpowering the happiness of survival, coping mechanisms are crucial. Support groups, counseling, and mindfulness practices provide comfort to a lot of survivors. It is essential to be open and honest with medical professionals regarding worries and symptoms to reduce worry and boost the survivor's self-assurance in their ability to adjust to life following treatment.

HONORING SIGNIFICANT OCCASIONS

Many significant events that occur along a person's journey are reasons to celebrate. Whether it's finishing treatment, marking a particular anniversary after diagnosis, or accomplishing personal objectives, survivors frequently find inspiration and strength in celebrating these victories.

There are many different ways to celebrate, from private get-togethers with loved ones to introspective analyses of the path taken. In addition to encouraging a sense of accomplishment, marking and celebrating milestones offers a chance for appreciation and introspection on the bravery and resiliency shown during the cancer journey.

After treatment, life is a complex path that includes developing a new sense of normalcy, healing on an emotional and physical level, and recovering physically.

The integration of survivor and follow-up care, continuous health monitoring, recurrence fear management, and milestone celebrations forms a comprehensive strategy for helping individuals navigate the distinct obstacles and victories of life following cancer treatment.

CHAPTER EIGHT

REPRODUCTIVE HEALTH AND FERTILITY

RECOGNIZING HOW UTERINE CANCER AFFECTS FERTILITY

Fertility can be severely impacted in those who have uterine cancer, a cancer that starts in the uterine tissues. The uterus, which is the organ in which the fertilized egg implants and develops into a fetus during pregnancy, is vital to the reproductive process. This complex mechanism can be interfered with when uterine cancer takes hold. Reproductive organs may unintentionally be damaged or removed as a result of the main therapies for uterine cancer, including radiation therapy, chemotherapy, and surgery. This can have an impact on fertility.

The effects of uterine cancer on fertility are frequently dual for women who are diagnosed with it. First off, hysterectomy, or surgical removal of the uterus, is a popular treatment for uterine cancer. Because of the absence of the necessary organ for gestation, this makes natural conception impossible. Second, the harshness of cancer therapies can damage the ovaries, decreasing their capacity and perhaps leading to early ovarian failure. Thus, the decreasing number of viable eggs further reduces the likelihood of conception.

For those impacted by uterine cancer, breakthroughs in assisted reproductive technologies provide hope despite these obstacles. In vitro fertilization (IVF) is one technique that can help people conceive using preserved eggs or embryos, depending on the situation and the stage of cancer diagnosis. But it's important to recognize the emotional toll that receiving a cancer diagnosis and the related infertility issues may have, underscoring the necessity of receiving thorough support and counseling at every step of the way.

OPTIONS FOR PRESERVING FERTILITY

The preservation of fertility has become a crucial factor for people whose health threatens their ability to procreate, such as those undergoing cancer treatments. Options for preserving fertility can give cancer patients a route to parenthood after therapy. Cryopreservation of eggs or embryos before cancer treatment is one such method.

Ocyte cryopreservation, often known as egg freezing, enables women to store their eggs for future use. To carry out this operation, the ovaries are stimulated to generate several eggs, which are then taken out, frozen, and kept until the person is ready to conceive. In contrast, embryo cryopreservation entails creating embryos by fertilizing eggs with sperm and then storing them for later use. These methods provide an opportunity to preserve fertility, particularly for those whose cancer treatments may impair it.

For men undergoing therapies that could endanger their fertility, sperm banking is a well-established alternative in addition to egg and embryo preservation. Sperm can be extracted, frozen, and kept for use in IVF and other assisted reproductive techniques in the future. Even amid difficult medical situations, people are empowered to make decisions about their reproductive destiny because of this proactive approach.

ADAPTING TO MODIFICATIONS IN REPRODUCTIVE HEALTH

Receiving a diagnosis of a disease that affects reproductive health, such as uterine cancer, can be emotionally and mentally taxing. Adapting to the shifts in reproductive health requires negotiating a challenging terrain of social, emotional, and physical ramifications.

It is recommended that people join support groups, seek counseling, or talk to their spouses about reproductive issues during this period because emotional support is crucial. To fully grasp your options and make an informed decision about fertility preservation or other family-building measures, be open with your healthcare providers.

Additionally, adopting a holistic perspective on well-being can make it easier to adjust to changes in reproductive health. This could entail making lifestyle adjustments that support general well-being and fertility, like eating a balanced diet, working out frequently, and controlling stress. Acupuncture and mindfulness exercises are examples of integrative therapies that can help maintain emotional stability during the difficult process of managing reproductive health and preserving fertility.

A thorough comprehension of the effects of uterine cancer on fertility, awareness of choices for fertility preservation, and practical coping mechanisms are essential elements of the path for those confronting these difficulties. People can handle the complexity of changes in reproductive health with resilience and optimism for the future by addressing these factors comprehensively.

CHAPTER NINE

AWARENESS AND ADVOCACY

BECOMING YOUR ADVOCATE

Encouraging people to actively engage in decisions about their health by empowering them to become their advocates is an important idea in the healthcare field. Within the context of healthcare, self-advocacy entails managing one's health, posing inquiries, and gathering data to enable well-informed choices. It is particularly relevant in circumstances when people can be given complicated diagnoses, such as uterine cancer. Fostering a proactive attitude toward healthcare, interacting with healthcare providers, and actively taking part in the decision-making process are all components of being your advocate.

Self-advocacy is more than just being able to communicate; it also includes knowing one's rights, getting second opinions, and accepting a cooperative relationship with medical professionals. Being an informed patient in the case of uterine cancer entails learning about the disease, available treatments, and any possible adverse effects. It also means speaking up, inquiring about complementary and alternative therapies, and making sure that individual beliefs and preferences are taken into account when making decisions. In the end, being your advocate means accepting responsibility for your health and collaborating with medical professionals to get the greatest results.

INCREASING AWARENESS OF UTERINE CANCER

Increasing awareness of uterine cancer is crucial for better outcomes, early identification, and the development of a community that supports people impacted by the illness. When compared to other malignancies, uterine cancer is frequently disregarded; therefore, public awareness campaigns on its warning signs, risk factors, and preventive measures need to be strengthened. Campaigns to raise awareness are essential for debunking misconceptions, lowering stigma, and promoting routine screenings.

Raising awareness involves using a variety of channels, such as social media, educational initiatives, and local gatherings. By reaching a large audience, these programs hope to educate women about the warning signs of uterine cancer and the value of getting help from a doctor as soon as possible. Raising awareness also involves campaigning for funds for research, since better preventative and treatment techniques can only be developed with a deeper understanding of the condition.

Developing a network of support for individuals impacted by uterine cancer is a crucial component of awareness initiatives. People can share their stories, offer emotional support, and improve the general well-being of persons facing the difficulties of uterine cancer by creating a feeling of community.

BOOSTING INNOVATION AND RESEARCH

It is critical to support uterine cancer research and advancements to improve patient outcomes, treatment options, and diagnostic techniques. Research serves as the basis for the creation of novel treatments, the enhancement of current therapies, and the comprehension of the fundamental causes of uterine cancer. In addition to soliciting funding, advocacy for research entails actively pushing laws that give priority to this kind of scientific investigation.

For uterine cancer research to advance more quickly, cooperation between researchers, medical professionals, and advocacy organizations is crucial. The scientific community can combine resources, exchange information, and accelerate the discovery of discoveries that could fundamentally alter the way uterine cancer is identified and treated by promoting interdisciplinary collaborations.

Public lobbying is essential in pushing policies that prioritize funding for research and make it easier for scientific discoveries to be translated into practical applications, in addition to providing financial assistance. Individuals and organizations can advance medical knowledge and improve outcomes for uterine cancer patients by lobbying for higher investment in the disease's research and interacting with lawmakers.